REAL

~~CONNECTIONS~~

Simplifying and Balancing - A New Blueprint for Raising Children.

PUBLISHED BY: CHOC PIE

Introduction

Parenting has always been a journey of learning, adapting, and growing alongside our children. But in today's world, we face an unprecedented challenge: raising kids in an era where social media is as pervasive as air. From the moment we share our first ultrasound photo online to our child's first steps, birthdays, or graduations, social media has become intertwined with the way we document, share, and even experience parenting.

On one hand, social media offers unparalleled benefits. It connects us with a global network of parents, providing advice, support, and a sense of community. We can find tips on sleep training, meal planning, or even how to handle tantrums with a simple scroll through Instagram or TikTok. But with these benefits come challenges. Social media often creates a highlight reel of parenting, showcasing picture-perfect families, spotless homes, and children who seem to excel at everything. It's easy to feel overwhelmed or inadequate, wondering if we're doing enough or measuring up.

Beyond the personal challenges, social media also raises ethical questions. How much should we share about our children online? What are the long-term implications of "sharenting"? And how can we ensure our kids grow up with a healthy relationship with technology and social media?

This book is about navigating the complex intersection of parenting and social media. It's not about demonizing technology or telling you to delete your accounts. Instead, it's about finding balance—using social media as a tool for connection and learning without letting it dictate our self-worth or parenting choices. It's about understanding the digital world so we can guide our children through it with confidence and clarity.

As you read through this book, you'll find practical strategies, real-life examples, and thought-provoking insights. Whether you're a new parent overwhelmed by the flood of online advice or a seasoned one navigating the challenges of raising teens in a hyper-connected world, this book aims to empower you to embrace intentional, mindful parenting in the age of social media.

Together, let's explore how we can raise strong, confident children while staying grounded in our values as parents. After all, the most important "likes" come from the people in your home—not the ones on your screen.

Contents

Contents

'The challenges'

Chapter 1: The Rise of Digital Parenting

Social media has fundamentally reshaped the way parents approach their roles, offering access to advice, support, and inspiration at our fingertips. For many, platforms like Instagram, TikTok, Facebook, and YouTube have become virtual parenting guides. On these platforms, parents can find everything from baby sleep-training techniques to lunchbox inspiration and parenting hacks.

The Positive Impact of Social Media

Social media has created opportunities for connection and community that didn't exist before. Parents can:

- **Access Immediate Advice**: From quick solutions to parenting dilemmas to tutorials on everyday challenges, social media provides a library of instant resources. For instance, a struggling parent can find expert advice on sleep training or creative meal ideas in minutes.

- **Find Community**: Virtual parenting groups bring together people from all over the world, offering a sense of camaraderie and mutual support. Whether it's a Facebook group for new mothers or an Instagram community focused on raising neurodivergent children, these networks help parents feel less isolated.

- **Share Experiences**: Social media allows parents to document milestones and share their joys and struggles with family, friends, and like-minded communities. This sharing can create a sense of validation and connection, reminding parents they are not alone in their journey.

The Role of Influencers

The rise of parenting influencers has added a new layer to the social media landscape. These "momfluencers" and "dadfluencers" often share relatable content that can validate a parent's feelings or offer innovative ideas. Influencers can:

- **Provide Inspiration**: Many influencers share creative parenting tips, educational activities, and hacks for simplifying daily routines, which can be incredibly helpful for busy parents.

- **Normalize Struggles**: Authentic influencers who share their challenges and imperfections can make other parents feel less alone in their struggles.

- **Shape Trends**: From sustainable baby products to parenting philosophies like gentle parenting, influencers often drive new trends in parenting.

However, influencers also set trends and standards that may not always be realistic for every family. The polished, curated nature of their content can create unrealistic expectations and pressure parents to strive for unattainable ideals.

The Hidden Challenges

While the benefits are clear, social media also brings challenges that can subtly undermine a parent's confidence or focus:

- **Information Overload**: The sheer volume of parenting advice online can overwhelm rather than clarify. Conflicting tips and methods can leave parents second-guessing their decisions.

- **Unrealistic Expectations**: Perfectly curated posts can make parents feel inadequate, as they compare their lives to idealized portrayals. A spotless home or a picture-perfect family dinner may not reflect the reality behind the scenes.

- **Judgment and Shaming**: Parenting choices often become topics of debate online, exposing parents to unsolicited criticism. This shaming can lead to guilt and self-doubt, even when parents are doing their best.

Navigating Digital Dependency

Many parents find themselves turning to social media for validation, whether through likes, comments, or views. This dependency can:

- **Shift Focus**: Parents may prioritize crafting shareable moments over being fully present with their children. The pressure to post the perfect photo or video can detract from genuine interactions.

- **Create Performance Anxiety**: The desire to "perform" parenting for an audience can overshadow the authentic experience of raising a child.

- **Fuel Comparison**: Constant exposure to idealized portrayals can lead to feelings of inadequacy, as parents compare their lives to influencers or peers.

To navigate these challenges, parents must develop a mindful approach to social media use, recognizing its benefits while setting boundaries to prevent it from overshadowing real-life connections. This chapter sets the stage for the rest of the book, helping parents recognize how social media has integrated itself into modern parenting and why it's essential to approach it with intention and mindfulness.

Checklist *Check ✓ if you do and ✗ if you don't*

1. **Understanding Your Digital Environment:**

- Do I know how much time my child spends on screens daily?

- Am I aware of the apps, websites, or platforms my child uses regularly?

- Have I observed how technology affects my child's behaviour, mood, or sleep patterns?

2. **Assessing My Digital Awareness as a Parent:**

- Do I stay updated on the latest digital trends, apps, and online platforms?

- Am I familiar with online safety risks (e.g., cyberbullying, privacy issues, inappropriate content)?

- Have I educated myself about parental control tools and settings?

3. **Setting a Family Digital Standard:**

- Do I model healthy screen use for my children?

- Have I discussed digital boundaries (like screen time limits) with my child?

- Is there an agreed-upon space and time where devices are not allowed (e.g., during meals or bedtime)?

Challenges *Check ✓ when you complete the challenges*

1. **Screen Time Audit:**

o   Track your child's screen use for one week (include time spent on phones, tablets, TV, and gaming).

o   Reflect on any patterns or surprises and identify areas for improvement.

2. **Family Digital Discussion:**

o   Have an open conversation with your child about their Favorite apps or online activities.

o   Ask questions like: "What do you enjoy most online?" or "What frustrates you about technology?"

3. **Technology-Free Zone Challenge:**

o   Designate one room in your home (e.g., the dining room) or one specific time (e.g., 8–9 PM) as a tech-free zone for the whole family.

o   Reflect on how this changes family interactions.

4. **Explore Parental Control Features:**

o   Spend 30 minutes setting up or reviewing parental controls on your child's devices.

o   Test one feature (e.g., screen time limits or app restrictions) to see how it works.

5. **Modelling Exercise:**

o   Identify one digital habit you can improve in your own life (e.g., reducing phone use during meals).

o   Share this change with your child and explain why you're doing it.

Chapter 2: The Pressure of Perfection

Parenting on social media often comes with an unspoken pressure to appear perfect. Platforms like Instagram, TikTok, and Pinterest are filled with curated posts that showcase spotless homes, well-behaved children, and beautifully staged family moments. These feeds often give the impression that successful parenting is always orderly, joyful, and aesthetically pleasing. Viral TikTok hacks and Instagram "reels" make it seem as though there's a quick fix for every challenge, from tantrums to meal prep. While these portrayals can be inspiring, they rarely reflect the chaos, struggles, and imperfection of real-life parenting, creating unrealistic expectations for parents who are simply trying their best.

The Myth of Effortless Parenting

Social media tends to glorify a version of parenting that appears flawless, presenting an unrealistic ideal that can feel unattainable. Posts and videos often focus on:

- **Perfectly Staged Moments**: Images of children reading quietly in spotless playrooms or eating healthy meals without complaint dominate social media feeds. These moments are often carefully curated, edited, and staged, giving the illusion that such behaviour is effortless and constant.

- **High-Achieving Milestones**: Parents frequently share posts about their children's academic or extracurricular successes, such as reading at an advanced level, excelling in sports, or achieving creative milestones. These posts rarely include the context of the hard work, struggles, or failures that often precede such achievements.

- **Idealized Family Dynamics**: Social media content often portrays harmonious family relationships where everyone is smiling, cooperating, and happy. Conflict, exhaustion, and moments of disconnection are conspicuously absent, perpetuating the idea that good parenting means avoiding struggles altogether.

These images promote the false notion that good parenting is easy and should always look picture-perfect. This can lead to feelings of inadequacy for parents whose daily realities include tantrums, messy homes, and the inevitable challenges of raising children. The gap between the polished portrayals on social media and the often-chaotic reality of parenting fosters unrealistic expectations and can make parents feel like they are failing simply because their lives don't match the ideal.

Recognizing the "Highlight Reel"

It's important to remember that social media often reflects a "highlight reel," not the full story. Behind every polished photo or viral video, there are untold struggles, messy moments, and hard work that remain unseen. The perfectly posed family photo may have required dozens of attempts, and the child reading quietly might have just finished a meltdown. Understanding this curated nature helps parents see beyond the surface and avoid internalizing the false perfection they perceive.

Moreover, many influencers and everyday users meticulously edit their content to align with trends or aesthetics, further masking the realities of parenting. Recognizing this can help parents put what they see online into perspective and remind them that their own imperfect moments are not failures but a natural part of parenting. It allows parents to focus on their authentic journey rather than striving for an unattainable ideal.

Real connections

Strategies to Resist the Comparison Trap

1. **Curate Your Feed**:

   - Follow accounts that promote authenticity and celebrate imperfect, real-life parenting. Seek out influencers who share the messy and meaningful parts of parenting, offering a more realistic and relatable perspective.

   - Unfollow or mute accounts that make you feel inadequate or overwhelmed. If a feed consistently triggers feelings of insecurity or self-doubt, it's okay to step back from it for the sake of your well-being.

2. **Focus on Your Wins**:

   - Reflect on your parenting strengths and the unique bond you have with your children. These strengths are what make your journey special and worth celebrating.

   - Celebrate small victories, like resolving a tantrum, managing a hectic day, or simply making your child smile. These moments, though small, reflect meaningful achievements in your parenting journey.

3. **Limit Screen Time**:

   - Reduce the time spent scrolling through social media, especially during moments of self-doubt or stress. Utilize tools such as app timers or screen usage trackers to help enforce these boundaries.

   - Replace screen time with activities that foster genuine connection with your family. Consider board games, outdoor play, or a dedicated family reading hour to strengthen real-life interactions.

4. **Practice Gratitude**:

o   Keep a journal to note three things you're grateful for in your parenting journey each day. This could be anything from a sweet moment with your child to a simple achievement like getting through the day's challenges.

o   Shift focus from comparison to appreciation for what you've achieved and experienced. Gratitude not only uplifts your perspective but also helps you recognize the value of your unique parenting path.

Changing the Narrative

Parents can play a pivotal role in reshaping the social media landscape by embracing and sharing authentic, unfiltered moments. By stepping away from the pressure to present a perfect image, parents can foster a more honest and supportive online environment that reflects the true highs and lows of raising children.

- **Share the Challenges**: Post about the messy days—the tantrums, the laundry piles, and the days when nothing seems to go as planned. These moments are universal among parents and can create a sense of solidarity and mutual understanding.

- **Celebrate Small Joys**: Highlight the little victories and everyday moments that make parenting rewarding. These can range from a quiet cuddle to a homemade craft that didn't go as planned but was fun anyway.

- **Encourage Real Conversations**: Use your platform to spark genuine dialogue about the realities of parenting. Ask questions, share insights, and engage with others to build a community that values connection over perfection.

By normalizing imperfection and celebrating the authenticity of the parenting journey, parents can challenge the curated highlight reels that dominate social media. This shift not only alleviates the pressure to conform but also creates a space where other parents feel seen, supported, and understood.

This chapter encourages readers to recognize the pressures social media creates, reframe their perspectives, and embrace the messy, beautiful reality of their own parenting journey. By doing so, they contribute to a digital culture that values authenticity over aesthetics and connection over comparison.

Checklist *Check ✓ if you do and ✗ if you don't*

1. Evaluating Digital Habits:

o   Have I identified digital habits (both positive and negative) that my child has developed?

o   Do I understand how my child's digital habits align with their overall wellbeing (e.g., academic, social, physical)?

2. Setting Boundaries:

o   Have I communicated clear digital rules and boundaries with my child?

o   Do I enforce consistent screen time limits across devices?

o   Have I created a balance between screen-based and non-screen activities?

3. Encouraging Responsible Digital Use:

o   Have I taught my child about the importance of digital etiquette (e.g., being respectful online)?

o   Have I explained privacy basics, such as not sharing personal information?

o   Do I encourage tech-free activities like outdoor play, reading, or hobbies?

4. Leading by Example:

o   Am I modelling balanced and mindful technology use in my daily life?

o   Do I avoid over-reliance on devices for entertainment or distractions?

Challenges *Check ✓ when you complete the challenges*

1. **Digital Habit Tracker:**

    o   Observe and record your child's digital habits for three days (e.g., screen time duration, preferred activities).
    o   Analyse whether these habits support or hinder their personal development.

2. **Create a Digital Contract:**

    o   Collaborate with your child to create a simple family digital use agreement.
    o   Include rules about screen time, device-free zones, and consequences for breaking the agreement.

3. **Encourage a Tech-Free Day:**

    o   Plan a tech-free day or a half-day where the entire family participates in offline activities.
    o   Reflect on how this impacts family dynamics and creativity.

4. **Teach Digital Etiquette:**

    o   Spend 15 minutes discussing with your child how to be respectful online (e.g., avoiding harmful comments, understanding cyberbullying).
    o   Role-play scenarios to practice digital manners.

5. **Introduce the "Digital Pause" Rule:**

    o   Establish a rule where family members pause before using their devices to reflect on why they're picking it up.
    o   Encourage your child to ask themselves: "Do I really need this now, or can I do something else?"

What small change can I make to help my child develop healthier digital habits?

How can I balance enforcing boundaries while respecting my child's growing independence?

Chapter 3: The "Sharenting" Dilemma

Parents are sharing more about their children online than ever before, but what are the consequences? The term "sharenting" refers to the act of parents sharing content about their children on social media. While it can be a way to celebrate milestones, connect with others, and document family life, sharenting also brings ethical and practical challenges that warrant careful consideration.

The Double-Edged Sword of Sharenting

Sharenting can have positive outcomes, such as fostering connections with extended family, friends, and supportive online communities. However, the practice also carries significant risks:

- **Privacy Concerns**: Every post about a child contributes to their digital footprint, which may include identifiable information such as names, locations, and activities. This information can be exploited by malicious actors or resurface in unintended contexts as the child grows.

- **Lack of Consent**: Young children are unable to consent to the content shared about them. As they age, they may feel uncomfortable or resentful about their digital presence created without their input.

- **Long-Term Implications**: Photos, videos, and anecdotes shared online can follow a child into adulthood, potentially impacting their relationships, education, or career prospects.

Questions to Consider Before Posting

To navigate the fine line between sharing meaningful moments and safeguarding a child's future, parents can ask themselves the following questions:

1. **Why Am I Sharing This?**

     o   Is the post meant to celebrate a milestone, seek advice, or connect with loved ones? Or is it motivated by external validation, such as likes and comments?

2. **Would My Child Approve?**

     o   How might your child feel about this content now and in the future? Would they be embarrassed, uncomfortable, or proud of what's being shared?

3. **Does This Post Reveal Too Much?**

     o   Avoid sharing details that could compromise your child's privacy or safety, such as school names, locations, or personal routines.

4. **Who Can See This?**

     o   Review your privacy settings to ensure the content is only visible to trusted individuals. Consider creating a private group for family updates.

Balancing Sharing and Safeguarding

Sharenting doesn't have to be all or nothing. Here are strategies to balance connection and privacy:

- **Opt for Limited Sharing**: Use private messaging or password-protected photo albums to share milestones with close friends and family instead of posting publicly.

- **Respect Your Child's Boundaries**: As children grow, involve them in decisions about what content is shared. Older kids may want to review or approve posts that include them.

- **Focus on Yourself**: Share parenting experiences and insights that centre on your journey rather than your child's personal details.

The Changing Legal and Social Landscape

As awareness of sharenting grows, so do conversations about its legal and ethical implications. Governments around the world are beginning to recognize the importance of safeguarding children's digital privacy. For instance, some countries are exploring legislation that would limit how much personal information parents can share about their children online without consent. These measures aim to protect children from potential exploitation and ensure they have greater control over their digital identities as they grow older.

Social media platforms are also stepping up to address these concerns by enhancing privacy features. Tools like audience restrictions, content moderation, and advanced parental controls allow users to better manage who can see their posts and what information is shared. However, these tools require active use, and many parents may not be fully aware of the options available to them.

In addition to legislative and technological developments, cultural attitudes are shifting. There is a growing movement among parents and advocacy groups to promote mindful sharing. This movement encourages families to prioritize children's consent and long-term well-being over the fleeting gratification of likes and comments. By staying informed about these trends and adapting to the evolving legal and social landscape, parents can make more conscious choices that respect their children's privacy and autonomy.

Creating a Sharenting Policy for Your Family

Developing a family policy for online sharing can provide clarity and consistency. Consider the following steps:

1. **Define Your Boundaries:**

   o   Decide what types of content are off-limits, such as bath time photos, tantrums, or anything overly personal.

2. **Set Age-Appropriate Guidelines:**

   o   Adjust sharing practices as your child grows, respecting their increasing autonomy and preferences.

3. **Regularly Review Your Practices:**

   o   Periodically revisit your family's approach to sharenting, ensuring it aligns with your values and your child's evolving needs.

Sharenting is a deeply personal decision, but one that carries lasting implications for children. By approaching it thoughtfully, parents can Honor their child's privacy while still celebrating the joys of parenting and connecting with their communities.

Checklist *Check ✓ if you do and ✗ if you don't*

1. **Building Open Communication:**

   o   Have I created an environment where my child feels comfortable discussing their digital experiences with me?

   o   Do I listen without judgement when my child shares online challenges or preferences?

2. **Co-Creating Digital Rules:**

   o   Have I involved my child in creating family digital rules (e.g., screen time, device-free zones)?

   o   Are the rules clear, fair, and age-appropriate?

3. **Encouraging Balanced Tech Use:**

   o   Do I encourage my child to balance online and offline activities (e.g., hobbies, outdoor play, and social interactions)?

   o   Have I discussed the importance of breaks from screens for mental and physical health?

4. **Setting Positive Screen Examples:**

   o   Am I modelling the digital habits I want my child to adopt (e.g., putting away devices during family time)?

   o   Do I avoid using technology as a "babysitter" or default solution for boredom?

5. **Reinforcing Positive Digital Experiences:**

   o   Have I praised or encouraged my child's positive digital behaviours, such as creating content or learning online?

   o   Do I focus on celebrating successes instead of only pointing out mistakes?

Challenges *Check ✓ when you complete the challenges*

1. **Family Digital Agreement:**

o   Sit down with your child and co-create a "family digital agreement."

o   Include rules for screen time, appropriate content, and shared responsibilities for staying safe online.

2. **Tech Time Alternatives:**

o   Work with your child to brainstorm non-digital activities they enjoy.

o   Plan at least one tech-free family activity each week (e.g., board games, nature walks).

3. **Practice Active Listening:**

o   Ask your child open-ended questions about their digital experiences (e.g., "What do you like most about this game/app?").

o   Avoid interrupting or offering immediate solutions—just listen and understand their perspective.

4. **Create a "Tech Positivity" Board:**

o   Collaborate with your child to list positive ways they can use technology (e.g., learning, creating, connecting with family).

o   Place this list somewhere visible as a reminder of healthy digital habits.

5. **Shared Digital Goal Challenge:**

o   Set a shared digital goal as a family (e.g., reducing unnecessary screen time by 30 minutes daily).

o   Track progress together and celebrate small wins.

How can I better involve my child in decisions about their digital habits?
What new insights did I gain from listening to my child's perspective on technology?

<u>'The Solution'</u>

Chapter 4: Modelling Healthy Social Media Habits

Children are like sponges—they absorb behaviours, habits, and attitudes from their parents. Every time you scroll through your phone, react to a notification, or share a post, your children are observing and learning. Whether it's how often you pick up your device, the tone of your interactions online, or how you handle feedback from others, these behaviours shape their understanding of what is normal and acceptable. Your relationship with social media serves as a template for theirs, making it essential to model healthy habits that demonstrate balance, intentionality, and mindful usage. By setting clear examples, you help your children navigate technology as a tool for growth and connection, rather than as a source of distraction or validation.

Understanding Your Influence

As a parent, your actions speak louder than words. Children are highly perceptive and form their attitudes toward technology based on how they see you use it. If your children frequently see you prioritising your phone over family time—answering emails at the dinner table, scrolling through social media during playtime, or reacting instantly to every notification—they may internalise the idea that screens hold greater importance than face-to-face interactions. This can inadvertently teach them that digital engagement is more rewarding than real-life connection.

On the other hand, when you use social media responsibly and with purpose, you model the positive role technology can play in a balanced life. For instance, using your phone to plan a family outing, share meaningful updates with loved ones, or learn new skills demonstrates how technology can be a valuable tool rather than a source of distraction. By showing your children that digital devices are a complement to—not a replacement for—real-world relationships, you set the foundation for them to develop healthy and intentional technology habits.

Setting Boundaries for Yourself

Modelling healthy habits begins with self-awareness. Reflect on how, when, and why you use social media, and recognise the potential impact of your behaviours on your children. By setting clear and intentional boundaries, you create a framework for healthier digital engagement that your children can emulate. Consider implementing these boundaries:

- **Designate Tech-Free Zones and Times**: Keep phones out of bedrooms and off the dining table to foster more meaningful family interactions. Tech-free zones create space for face-to-face conversations, deeper connections, and undistracted engagement.

- **Schedule Downtime**: Set aside specific periods to step away from devices, such as during morning routines or an hour before bedtime. This not only improves focus and mental clarity but also models the importance of balance between digital and real-world activities.

- **Limit Notifications**: Turn off non-essential alerts to reduce distractions and stay present in the moment. Managing notifications helps you prioritise what matters most, ensuring that your attention is directed towards your family rather than unnecessary digital interruptions.

By consistently enforcing these boundaries, you demonstrate the value of mindful technology use and the importance of creating space for genuine connections within your home.

Demonstrating Intentional Use

Show your children how to use social media intentionally rather than passively, emphasising the importance of purpose and mindfulness. Demonstrating intentional use helps children understand that technology can be a tool for growth, connection, and learning when used thoughtfully. For example:

- **Use Social Media for Connection**: Demonstrate how to connect meaningfully with friends and family by sharing updates, engaging in thoughtful conversations, and celebrating milestones together. Explain how this builds real relationships instead of scrolling aimlessly.

- **Share Purposeful Content**: Encourage sharing posts that align with your values and goals. For example, share educational articles, creative projects, or inspirational stories rather than seeking external validation through likes or comments.

- **Learn and Grow Through Technology**: Use online communities and platforms as a resource for learning new skills or exploring hobbies. For instance, follow tutorials, join interest-based groups, or participate in virtual workshops. This shows children that social media can be more than just entertainment—it can be a gateway to personal and intellectual growth.

By consistently demonstrating these practices, you help children develop a mindset that values quality over quantity in their social media interactions, fostering a healthier and more intentional relationship with technology.

Real connections

Encouraging Balance

Balance is key to maintaining a healthy relationship with social media. It's important to emphasise that while technology has its benefits, it should never replace real-life connections and activities. Begin by discussing the significance of offline experiences and how they contribute to mental well-being, creativity, and stronger family bonds.

Actively participate in offline activities as a family to demonstrate the value of stepping away from screens. Schedule regular family outings such as trips to the park, hikes, or visits to museums. Create designated times for tech-free interactions, such as game nights, reading sessions, or family meals, where everyone can focus on each other without the distraction of devices.

Encourage your children to explore face-to-face interactions with friends, engage in outdoor play, and develop creative hobbies like drawing, writing, or building projects. Highlight the joys of these experiences and how they foster skills and memories that digital entertainment cannot replicate. By consistently promoting a balanced approach, you set a foundation for a healthier, more intentional relationship with technology.

Admitting and Correcting Mistakes

No one is perfect, and children benefit immensely from seeing their parents recognise and address their own mistakes. Admitting when you've overused your phone, been distracted during an important moment, or mismanaged your social media time teaches your children that mistakes are a natural part of life and an opportunity for growth.

When you catch yourself overusing your phone or allowing social media to intrude on family time, acknowledge it openly. For instance, you might say, "I realise I've been checking my phone too much during dinner. I'm sorry, and I'll make an effort to focus on our time together." This act of vulnerability shows your children the importance of self-awareness and accountability.

Taking corrective actions, like setting specific times to step away from devices or creating reminders to stay present, reinforces your commitment to improvement. Discussing these changes with your children further solidifies the lesson that everyone has the capacity to reflect, learn, and grow. This not only strengthens your bond but also models resilience and adaptability, qualities your children can emulate in their own lives.

Fostering Open Dialogue

Talking to your children about the purpose and effects of social media is one of the most effective ways to help them develop a healthy relationship with technology. Start by sharing your own thoughts and experiences with social media, highlighting both the benefits and the challenges it presents. For instance, discuss how you use social media to stay connected with friends or learn new things, but also acknowledge the distractions or pressures you face.

Encourage your children to ask questions or express their opinions about social media. Be open to listening without judgment, allowing them to share their feelings or frustrations about their online experiences. Questions like, "How do you feel after spending time on social media?" or "What do you think makes a post or comment positive or negative?" can spark meaningful discussions.

Create a safe space where your children feel comfortable coming to you with concerns about their online interactions. If they encounter cyberbullying, peer pressure, or troubling content, they should know they can trust you to support them without overreacting. These conversations not only build trust but also help children develop critical thinking skills and emotional awareness about their social media use.

By fostering open dialogue, you show your children that communication is key to navigating the digital world. You also lay the groundwork for them to approach technology responsibly, maintaining balance and purpose in both their digital and real-world lives.

Checklist *Check ✓ if you do and ✗ if you don't*

1. **Understanding Online Risks:**

   o   Do I know the most common online risks my child might face (e.g., cyberbullying, inappropriate content, scams)?

   o   Have I educated my child about these risks in an age-appropriate way?

2. **Teaching Critical Thinking:**

   o   Have I explained how to identify misinformation or scams online?

   o   Do I encourage my child to question online content and verify sources before believing or sharing information?

3. **Building Emotional Resilience:**

   o   Have I had conversations about how to respond to negativity online (e.g., unkind comments or exclusion)?

   o   Do I encourage my child to talk to me or a trusted adult if something online makes them uncomfortable?

4. **Online Privacy and Security:**

   o   Have I taught my child the importance of protecting personal information online?

   o   Do I regularly review privacy settings with them on their devices and social media accounts?

5. **Responding to Challenges:**

o   Am I prepared to support my child if they experience a negative online incident?

o   Have I outlined steps they can take to report or block harmful content or users?

Challenges *Check ✓ when you complete the challenges*

1. **Role-Playing Scenarios:**

    o   Act out common online risk scenarios with your child, such as encountering a mean comment or spotting a phishing email.
    o   Practice how they should respond and discuss why those steps are important.

2. **Teach "Stop, Think, Act":**

    o   Encourage your child to pause before sharing or engaging with online content.
    o   Use this three-step rule: "Stop" (pause to reflect), "Think" (consider the impact), "Act" (decide responsibly).

3. **Misinformation Hunt:**

    o   Explore online articles or social media posts together, identifying red flags for misinformation (e.g., clickbait titles, lack of credible sources).
    o   Teach them how to fact-check information using trusted sources.

4. **Online Privacy Check-Up:**

    o   Spend 30 minutes reviewing your child's device and social media privacy settings together.
    o   Explain what each setting does and why it's essential to protect personal data.

5. **Digital Support Plan:**

    o   Create a step-by-step plan for your child to follow if they encounter a negative online experience (e.g., block/report the user, take a screenshot, tell a trusted adult).
    o   Role-play using this plan for different situations.

What online risks does my child face most often, and how can I better prepare them to handle these? How can I ensure my child feels supported in sharing their digital challenges with me?

CHOC PIE

Chapter 5: Teaching Digital Literacy to Your Kids

The ability to navigate the digital world critically and responsibly is an essential skill for children today. With an overwhelming amount of information available online, teaching digital literacy has become as important as traditional education. This chapter focuses on empowering your child with the tools they need to make informed decisions, identify credible sources, understand the impact of algorithms, and practice online safety.

Recognizing Credible Sources

One of the most important aspects of digital literacy is the ability to evaluate the credibility of online content. Teach your child to:

- **Check the Source**: Encourage them to verify the credibility of the website or organisation providing the information. Reliable sources are usually associated with established institutions like universities, government agencies, or reputable news outlets.

- **Cross-Check Information**: Show them how to compare information across multiple sources to ensure accuracy.

- **Recognise Bias**: Discuss how content creators may have biases or agendas that shape their content, whether it's political, commercial, or personal.

Understanding the Impact of Algorithms

Algorithms influence much of what we see online, from social media feeds to search engine results. Help your child understand how algorithms work and why they might shape their online experience. For example:

- **Personalisation**: Explain how algorithms customise content based on past behaviour, such as likes, shares, or search history.

- **Echo Chambers**: Discuss the risks of being exposed to only one perspective and the importance of seeking diverse viewpoints.

- **Critical Engagement**: Encourage them to question why certain posts or ads appear and to think critically about the intent behind them.

Practicing Online Safety

Online safety is a cornerstone of digital literacy. Equip your child with the knowledge to protect themselves and their information:

- **Create Strong Passwords**: Teach them to use unique and complex passwords and explain the importance of not sharing them.

- **Avoid Oversharing**: Help them understand the risks of sharing personal information, such as their location, school, or daily routines.

- **Identify Red Flags**: Teach them to recognise phishing attempts, suspicious links, and scams.

- **Privacy Settings**: Show them how to adjust privacy settings on social media platforms to control who can see their content.

Encouraging Responsible Online Behaviour

Digital literacy isn't just about recognising risks; it's also about fostering positive behaviours. Encourage your child to:

- **Think Before Posting**: Remind them that anything shared online can have long-term consequences. Encourage thoughtful posting that reflects their values and respects others.
- **Respect Others**: Discuss the importance of being kind and respectful in online interactions, including how to handle disagreements constructively.
- **Limit Screen Time**: Promote a healthy balance between online and offline activities to ensure they're not overly reliant on digital devices.

By equipping your child with these skills, you empower them to navigate the digital world with confidence, curiosity, and caution. Digital literacy is an ongoing journey, but with the right guidance, children can become savvy, responsible, and ethical digital citizens.

Checklist *Check ✓ if you do and ✗ if you don't*

1. **Exploring Digital Creativity:**

   o   Have I identified my child's interests or passions that can be explored through digital tools (e.g., art, coding, music)?

   o   Do I provide access to safe and age-appropriate apps or platforms for creative expression?

2. **Encouraging Positive Online Engagement:**

   o   Have I discussed the importance of kindness and respect in online interactions?

   o   Do I encourage my child to use technology to connect positively with others (e.g., sharing ideas, collaborating on projects)?

3. **Balancing Creation and Consumption:**

   o   Do I encourage my child to spend time creating content rather than just consuming it (e.g., making videos, writing stories, designing games)?

   o   Have I set boundaries to ensure a balance between creative screen time and offline activities?

4. **Promoting Digital Responsibility:**

   o   Have I taught my child to credit sources and avoid plagiarism in their digital creations?

   o   Do I encourage discussions about the impact of their online actions and how they represent themselves digitally?

5. **Celebrating Achievements:**

   o   Do I acknowledge and celebrate my child's creative efforts and online contributions?

   o   Have I provided opportunities for them to share their creations with friends or family?

Challenges *Check ✓ when you complete the challenges*

1. **Creative Tech Project:**

   o   Encourage your child to start a creative digital project (e.g., designing a website, creating a digital scrapbook, or recording a podcast).

   o   Set aside time to explore and support their project together.

2. **Kindness Challenge:**

   o   Encourage your child to spread positivity online by writing a thoughtful comment, sharing something helpful, or creating content that inspires others.

   o   Reflect on how this makes them feel about their online presence.

3. **Introduce New Tools:**

   o   Explore a new creative digital tool together (e.g., a photo editing app, a coding platform, or music-making software).

   o   Let your child experiment with it to spark their interest in creating.

4. **Digital Creation Showcase:**

   o   Set up a "show-and-tell" session where your child shares something they've created digitally.

   o   Invite family members or friends to celebrate their effort and creativity.

5. **Positive Role Model Exercise:**

   o   Ask your child to identify a positive online role model or creator they admire.

   o   Discuss why they inspire them and how they can apply similar values or behaviours in their own digital activities.

Chapter 6: Building Emotional Resilience

Social media can amplify feelings of inadequacy and comparison, even for children. Constant exposure to idealised images, exaggerated successes, and curated content can make children question their own worth or feel as though they don't measure up. In a world where likes, shares, and comments can seem like measures of self-worth, it's vital to help children develop emotional resilience to navigate the digital landscape confidently. Emotional resilience equips children to face online challenges with self-assurance and clarity, enabling them to focus on their intrinsic value rather than seeking validation from external sources. This chapter highlights the importance of fostering self-worth, handling online criticism constructively, and building meaningful connections that go beyond superficial metrics.

Understanding the Impact of Social Media on Emotional Well-Being

Children are naturally impressionable, and social media often exposes them to a flood of unrealistic beauty standards, idealised lifestyles, and constant comparisons. Platforms filled with carefully curated posts can make it difficult for children to distinguish between reality and filtered portrayals, leading to distorted perceptions of success, happiness, and self-worth. These influences, if unchecked, can result in feelings of inadequacy, anxiety, and low self-esteem, as children begin to measure themselves against an impossible standard.

Without proper guidance, children may internalise the belief that their lives should mirror the perfection they see online. This can erode their confidence and make them overly reliant on external validation. Helping children recognise that social media content is often curated and not a true reflection of reality is a crucial first step in building resilience. By teaching them to question what they see and embrace their unique qualities, parents can empower children to develop a healthy sense of self-worth and emotional strength.

Strategies to Handle Online Criticism

1. **Normalise Imperfection**: Teach children that no one is perfect, and everyone makes mistakes. Highlight examples from your own life to show them how imperfection is a natural part of growth. This understanding can help them view criticism as an opportunity to improve rather than a personal attack. Normalising mistakes also reduces their fear of failure, allowing them to engage with the digital world more confidently.

2. **Focus on the Positive**: Encourage your child to pay attention to supportive and uplifting interactions. Help them understand that the internet is filled with a mix of constructive feedback and negativity, and choosing to focus on positivity can significantly improve their experience. Teach them to value praise and kind comments from trusted sources while learning to disregard negativity from strangers or unconstructive critics.

3. **Practice Constructive Response**: Role-play scenarios where your child might encounter online criticism. Guide them on how to evaluate whether a comment is constructive or harmful. For constructive criticism, teach them to respond thoughtfully, thanking the commenter if appropriate. For harmful comments, demonstrate how to either ignore, block, or report the individual while maintaining their composure. Practicing these scenarios builds confidence and prepares them to handle real-life situations calmly and effectively.

Building Confidence

- **Celebrate Strengths**: Regularly remind your child of their unique talents, skills, and qualities. Highlight specific examples, such as their creativity in art, their kindness toward friends, or their determination in school projects. Celebrate their achievements, both big and small, to reinforce a sense of pride and self-worth.

Building their confidence offline helps them feel secure about themselves online, making them less reliant on external validation.

- **Encourage Personal Goals**: Help children focus on their personal growth and achievements by setting realistic and meaningful goals. For instance, support them in improving a skill they enjoy, such as playing a musical instrument or excelling in a sport. Celebrate their progress and emphasise the value of effort and perseverance over external recognition like likes or comments. This approach fosters a sense

- of accomplishment and intrinsic motivation.

- **Limit Comparison**: Teach children to focus on their own journey rather than comparing themselves to others. Discuss how everyone's strengths, challenges, and circumstances differ, making comparisons both unfair and unproductive. Encourage them to appreciate their individuality and to view others' successes as inspiration rather than a source of insecurity. Role-play scenarios where they might feel the urge to compare and brainstorm positive ways to shift their mindset.

Fostering Meaningful Connections

- **Prioritise Offline Relationships**: Encourage your child to strengthen their bonds with friends and family through face-to-face interactions, which provide deeper and more authentic connections. Organise family activities such as game nights, outdoor adventures, or cooking together to nurture these relationships. Highlight the value of in-person experiences that foster trust and understanding beyond what digital connections can offer.

- **Teach Empathy Online**: Discuss the importance of being kind and supportive in online interactions. Role-play scenarios where they can practice responding to others with empathy, such as offering encouragement to a friend or standing up against negative comments. Teach them how empathy can transform digital spaces into more positive and inclusive environments.

- **Encourage Community Participation**: Help your child find online groups or communities that align with their interests, such as hobby forums, study groups, or social causes they care about. Emphasise collaboration and mutual support over competition. For example, encourage them to contribute to group projects or volunteer opportunities, showcasing how digital communities can be a force for good.

By focusing on these strategies, you empower your child to navigate the digital world with confidence and self-assurance, ensuring they value their intrinsic worth over fleeting metrics of online approval. Encourage them to balance digital and real-world connections, fostering a holistic approach to building meaningful relationships.

Checklist *Check ✓ if you do and ✗ if you don't*

1. **Exploring Digital Creativity:**
   - Have I identified my child's interests or passions that can be explored through digital tools (e.g., art, coding, music)?
   - Do I provide access to safe and age-appropriate apps or platforms for creative expression?

2. **Encouraging Positive Online Engagement:**
   - Have I discussed the importance of kindness and respect in online interactions?
   - Do I encourage my child to use technology to connect positively with others (e.g., sharing ideas, collaborating on projects)?

3. **Balancing Creation and Consumption:**
   - Do I encourage my child to spend time creating content rather than just consuming it (e.g., making videos, writing stories, designing games)?
   - Have I set boundaries to ensure a balance between creative screen time and offline activities?

4. **Promoting Digital Responsibility:**
   - Have I taught my child to credit sources and avoid plagiarism in their digital creations?
   - Do I encourage discussions about the impact of their online actions and how they represent themselves digitally?

5. **Celebrating Achievements:**
   - Do I acknowledge and celebrate my child's creative efforts and online contributions?
   - Have I provided opportunities for them to share their creations with friends or family?

Challenges *Check ✓ when you complete the challenges*

1. **Creative Tech Project:**
o   Encourage your child to start a creative digital project (e.g., designing a website, creating a digital scrapbook, or recording a podcast).
o   Set aside time to explore and support their project together.

2. **Kindness Challenge:**
o   Encourage your child to spread positivity online by writing a thoughtful comment, sharing something helpful, or creating content that inspires others.
o   Reflect on how this makes them feel about their online presence.

3. **Introduce New Tools:**
o   Explore a new creative digital tool together (e.g., a photo editing app, a coding platform, or music-making software).
o   Let your child experiment with it to spark their interest in creating.

4. **Digital Creation Showcase:**
o   Set up a "show-and-tell" session where your child shares something they've created digitally.
o   Invite family members or friends to celebrate their effort and creativity.

5. **Positive Role Model Exercise:**
o   Ask your child to identify a positive online role model or creator they admire.
o   Discuss why they inspire them and how they can apply similar values or behaviours in their own digital activities.

Chapter 7: Creating a Healthy Digital Environment

A healthy digital environment fosters balance and intentionality, helping families navigate technology without letting it dominate their lives. In today's hyperconnected world, devices have become a constant presence, often intruding on personal time, blurring boundaries between work and leisure, and diminishing the quality of family interactions. This over-reliance on technology can lead to increased stress, reduced face-to-face communication, and even feelings of isolation within the family unit.

Creating a healthy digital environment involves more than just setting limits; it requires a conscious effort to integrate technology thoughtfully into daily life while prioritising meaningful connections and activities. This chapter provides actionable steps to establish harmony between the digital and real worlds, empowering families to embrace the benefits of technology

while safeguarding their relationships and well-being.

Establishing Tech-Free Zones

Designate specific areas in your home where technology use is off-limits. These zones encourage face-to-face communication and foster meaningful connections:

- **The Dining Table**: Make mealtimes a tech-free experience, allowing everyone to share their day and strengthen family bonds.
- **Bedrooms**: Keep devices out of sleeping areas to promote better sleep hygiene and minimise distractions before bedtime.
- **Living Rooms During Quality Time**: Set aside times when the family can gather for activities like games, movies, or conversations without interruptions from phones or tablets.

CHOC PIE

Creating Family Agreements on Technology Use

Family agreements ensure everyone is on the same page about technology expectations. Involve your children in creating these guidelines to foster a sense of ownership and responsibility:

- **Set Time Limits**: Agree on daily screen time limits for both work and leisure activities, ensuring enough time is left for offline pursuits.

- **Define Appropriate Content**: Discuss what types of apps, games, and websites are suitable for each family member, tailoring rules to age and maturity.

- **Respect Shared Time**: Establish rules about not using devices during family activities or conversations.

Encouraging Meaningful Offline Interactions

Technology can enhance our lives, but it's essential to prioritise offline connections. Encourage activities that bring the family together and stimulate creativity and joy:

- **Plan Regular Tech-Free Days**: Dedicate one day a week to tech-free family activities like hiking, cooking, or visiting local attractions.

- **Promote Shared Hobbies**: Explore interests such as gardening, crafting, or sports that encourage collaboration and interaction.

- **Foster Open Communication**: Use tech-free moments to discuss hopes, challenges, and goals as a family, reinforcing trust and understanding.

Balancing Digital Benefits with Boundaries

While boundaries are important, embracing the positive aspects of technology is equally vital. For example:

- **Educational Tools**: Incorporate apps and platforms that promote learning and skill-building for children and adults alike.

- **Family Digital Projects**: Work on a creative digital activity together, such as making a family photo album or creating a video journal.

- **Staying Connected**: Use technology to maintain ties with distant relatives and friends through video calls and shared updates.

By implementing these strategies, you create an environment where technology is a tool to enhance life rather than dominate it. A healthy digital environment sets the stage for children to develop balanced habits and ensures that family relationships thrive in a connected world.

Checklist *Check ✓ if you do and ✗ if you don't*

1. **Identifying Conflict Triggers:**
   - Do I recognise common triggers for technology-related conflicts in my family (e.g., excessive screen time, inappropriate content)?
   - Have I considered how my own digital habits might contribute to these conflicts?

2. **Setting Clear Expectations:**
   - Have I clearly communicated our family's digital boundaries and expectations?
   - Do I involve my child in creating these expectations to ensure they feel heard?

3. **Practising Calm Conflict Resolution:**
   - Do I address tech-related issues calmly and without judgement?
   - Have I established strategies for resolving disagreements about digital use?

4. **Fostering Positive Digital Relationships:**
   - Do I encourage my child to build respectful and meaningful online relationships?
   - Have I taught them how to recognise and handle unhealthy online interactions (e.g., trolling, toxic friendships)?

5. **Reviewing and Adjusting:**
   - Do I regularly review our family's digital rules to ensure they remain relevant as my child grows?
   - Have I provided opportunities for my child to share their thoughts or concerns about digital use?

Challenges *Check ✓ when you complete the challenges*

1. **Conflict Reflection Exercise:**

- Identify one recent technology-related conflict in your family. Reflect on:
    - o What triggered the conflict?
    - o How was it handled?
    - o What could have been done differently to resolve it peacefully?

2. **Family Tech Meeting:**

o Host a family meeting to discuss digital rules and expectations.

o Encourage everyone to share their views and propose solutions for recurring tech-related issues.

3. **Teach Healthy Digital Relationship Skills:**

o Role-play scenarios with your child on handling difficult online interactions (e.g., responding to mean comments, ending toxic friendships).

o Discuss ways to build positive connections, such as supporting friends online.

4. **Model Conflict Management:**

o Commit to addressing technology-related issues calmly and constructively.

o Practice stating your concerns without blame and offering solutions that involve your child's input.

5. **Revisit Digital Agreements:**

o Review your family's digital rules or agreements with your child.

o Adjust them based on your child's growing needs and your observations.

Chapter 8: Leveraging Social Media Positively

Social media isn't inherently harmful—it's a tool that, when used intentionally, can empower and inspire both parents and children. Its ability to connect individuals across the globe, share ideas, and foster creativity makes it a valuable resource for growth and enrichment. Whether it's discovering supportive communities, learning new skills, or showcasing creative projects, social media offers unique opportunities for families to thrive in the digital age. However, the key to unlocking its potential lies in using it thoughtfully, ensuring it enhances rather than detracts from our lives. This chapter delves into strategies for leveraging social media's strengths, fostering a balanced approach, and minimising its potential drawbacks to make it a positive force for both parents and children.

Accessing Supportive Communities

Social media provides a platform for parents to connect with others who share similar experiences, challenges, and interests. These online networks can be transformative in building relationships, gaining knowledge, and finding a sense of belonging:

- **Parenting Groups**: Online communities tailored to specific parenting needs can provide invaluable support. Whether you are a new parent seeking advice on baby care, raising a child with disabilities, or navigating the challenges of adolescence, these groups offer a space to share experiences, ask questions, and receive encouragement. Parenting groups often become a source of practical tips and emotional support, helping parents feel less isolated.

- **Learning Opportunities**: Social media is a hub for educational resources and evidence-based advice. Through forums, dedicated groups, and professional pages, parents can access a wealth of information on topics ranging from child development to creative activities. Many of these groups share step-by-step guides, video tutorials, and expert advice, making it easier for parents to learn and implement new ideas at home.

- **Shared Experiences**: Engaging with parents worldwide opens doors to diverse perspectives and experiences. Sharing stories of triumphs and struggles fosters a sense of camaraderie and understanding, reminding parents that they are not alone in their journey. These connections can provide a fresh outlook and offer creative solutions to common parenting challenges, building a global network of support and solidarity.

By tapping into these supportive communities, parents can gain confidence, broaden their horizons, and create meaningful relationships that enrich their parenting journey.

Sharing Meaningful Content

Social media offers an outlet for parents to share their unique experiences and values, contributing to a more authentic and positive digital landscape. When approached thoughtfully, sharing content can inspire others, promote important causes, and model responsible online behaviour for children:

- **Promote Positivity**: Share posts that uplift and inspire others. Highlight meaningful family moments, milestones, or lessons learned from challenges. For example, a post about a family activity that brought joy or a personal insight on navigating a parenting hurdle can resonate deeply with others and spread positivity.

- **Advocate for Causes**: Use your platform to draw attention to issues or organisations that align with your family's values. Whether it's advocating for environmental sustainability, mental health awareness, or community volunteerism, sharing these causes teaches children the importance of using their voice to make a difference responsibly and constructively.

- **Balance Authenticity and Privacy**: While it's valuable to share authentic content, ensure it respects your child's boundaries and privacy. Avoid oversharing details that could compromise their security or future comfort. For example, consider sharing broader parenting experiences rather than intimate details about your child's personal life, modelling mindful digital behaviour.

Fostering Creativity and Growth

Social media can be a powerful catalyst for creativity and intellectual development when used as a tool rather than a distraction. By leveraging its potential thoughtfully, parents can help children unlock new skills, collaborate on meaningful projects, and build confidence in their accomplishments:

- **Explore Creative Platforms**: Encourage children to engage with apps and platforms that inspire creativity and learning. For instance, platforms like Scratch can introduce coding in a fun and accessible way, while apps like Procreate enable children to explore digital art. Music-focused tools like GarageBand allow young minds to compose and experiment with sounds, nurturing their creative potential.

- **Collaborative Projects**: Use social media as an opportunity for family collaboration. Create a family blog documenting your adventures, produce short videos showcasing your cooking or DIY projects, or design a digital scrapbook highlighting family milestones. These activities not only foster creativity but also strengthen family bonds through shared goals and teamwork.

- **Celebrate Achievements**: Share your child's milestones and creative successes on social media in a way that promotes pride and motivation. For example, showcase their artwork, highlight a science project they completed, or share a short video of them performing a musical piece. This recognition reinforces the value of effort and persistence, building their confidence while teaching them to celebrate their unique talents.

By focusing on these strategies, social media becomes a tool for growth and innovation, empowering children to use technology as a means of self-expression and discovery rather than mere consumption.

Setting Boundaries for Positive Use

To ensure social media remains a positive influence, establish boundaries that encourage mindful engagement. These boundaries not only promote intentional use but also help maintain a healthy balance between the digital and real world:

- **Limit Consumption**: Encourage purposeful engagement with social media by focusing on creating or contributing rather than passively consuming content. For example, children and parents can work together on a family project, such as creating a photo album or crafting a positive post about a shared hobby. Limiting time spent mindlessly scrolling reduces exposure to negative influences and boosts productivity.

- **Curate Your Feed**: Be selective about the accounts you follow. Choose profiles that inspire and educate, such as those promoting creativity, wellness, or learning opportunities. Simultaneously, unfollow or mute accounts that trigger comparison, negativity, or anxiety. Regularly reviewing and updating your feed ensures it aligns with your personal and family values, creating a more uplifting and constructive online experience.

- **Encourage Reflection**: Initiate conversations with children about the difference between constructive and superficial content. Discuss how some posts are designed to mislead or evoke envy, while others genuinely inform or inspire. Foster a critical approach to social media consumption, helping children understand the intent behind what they see and empowering them to engage thoughtfully.

By leveraging the power of social media thoughtfully, parents and children can harness its potential to connect, inspire, and grow. This intentional approach transforms social media from a source of stress into a meaningful tool for personal and family enrichment.

Checklist *Check ✓ if you do and ✗ if you don't*

1. **Understanding Digital Independence:**

   o Have I assessed whether my child is ready for more online freedom based on their age, maturity, and behaviour?
   o Do I understand the online platforms, tools, or social media my child wants to use independently?

2. **Teaching Digital Responsibility:**

   o Have I taught my child the importance of managing their online reputation and digital footprint?
   o Do they understand how to protect their privacy and personal information online?
   o Have I discussed the risks of oversharing and the permanence of digital content?

3. **Encouraging Safe Decision-Making:**

   o Have I prepared my child to make safe decisions online without constant supervision?
   o Do they know how to identify and respond to online risks, such as phishing scams, inappropriate content, or cyberbullying?

4. **Building Trust and Accountability:**

   o Have I established clear expectations and consequences for their online behaviour?
   o Do I check in regularly to review their online experiences without micromanaging?

5. **Monitoring vs. Freedom:**

   o Do I use monitoring tools sparingly and openly discuss their purpose with my child?
   o Have I gradually reduced supervision as my child demonstrates responsible behaviour?

Challenges *Check ✓ when you complete the challenges*

1. **Digital Independence Readiness Assessment:**
o   Reflect on your child's current digital habits and maturity.
o   Identify areas where they need more guidance before granting additional freedom.

2. **Digital Footprint Review:**
o   Sit with your child to review their current online presence (e.g., social media profiles, shared posts).
o   Discuss how their digital footprint might be perceived by others and what changes they might consider.

3. **Online Safety Drill:**
o   Create hypothetical online scenarios (e.g., receiving a suspicious link, dealing with inappropriate messages) and ask your child how they would respond.
o   Provide feedback and reinforce safe decision-making practices.

4. **Responsibility Contract:**
o   Work with your child to create a digital responsibility contract outlining expectations for their online behaviour.
o   Include guidelines for privacy, respectful communication, and screen time limits.

5. **Gradual Freedom Plan:**
o   Develop a step-by-step plan for increasing your child's digital independence.
o   Start with small freedoms (e.g., managing their own screen time) and build up to larger responsibilities (e.g., using social media unsupervised).

Chapter 9: Encouraging Offline Family Connections

True connection often happens when devices are set aside, creating space for genuine interaction, empathy, and quality time. In a world increasingly dominated by screens, fostering offline connections is not just a luxury but a necessity for nurturing strong family bonds and building lasting memories. Offline interactions allow families to fully engage with one another, share experiences, and build trust without the distractions of notifications or digital interruptions. This chapter explores practical strategies for making offline time meaningful and enjoyable for every family member, offering a path toward deeper relationships and a sense of togetherness in an increasingly digital age.

The Importance of Being Present

When family members put away their devices, they open the door to deeper conversations, stronger emotional connections, and shared experiences. Being present goes beyond merely occupying the same space—it means actively engaging with one another, listening intently, and showing genuine interest in each other's thoughts and feelings. It's about creating moments of connection that build trust, empathy, and understanding within the family unit.

Prioritising presence encourages a sense of belonging and strengthens emotional bonds. It helps family members feel valued and heard, reducing feelings of isolation or neglect that can arise when attention is divided. By setting aside distractions like notifications or digital obligations, families can cultivate an atmosphere where every member feels seen and appreciated. These intentional moments of presence foster a positive family dynamic and create lasting memories that no device can replicate.

Practical Ways to Strengthen Bonds

- **Shared Meals**: Establish a tradition of eating together without screens. Use mealtimes as a sanctuary for connection, where everyone can share stories, discuss highlights of the day, or plan upcoming family activities. Enhance these moments by introducing themes like "International Cuisine Night" or inviting each family member to cook their favourite dish, turning meals into a collaborative and enjoyable experience.

- **Outdoor Adventures**: Organise nature walks, picnics, or hikes that encourage exploration, teamwork, and physical activity. Consider geocaching as a fun way to combine technology and adventure, or start a nature journal where each family member can document their discoveries. The natural environment provides a refreshing break from digital distractions and fosters an appreciation for the beauty of the world around us.

- **Creative Family Projects**: Collaborate on projects like building a garden, crafting, or cooking new recipes together. Turn these activities into long-term traditions, such as designing seasonal decorations, growing a family vegetable patch, or creating scrapbooks filled with cherished memories. These projects not only develop skills but also create opportunities for meaningful collaboration and a sense of shared accomplishment.

Meaningful Conversations

- **Daily Check-Ins**: Set aside time each day for a family check-in where everyone can share their thoughts, challenges, and successes. This can be as simple as sitting together after dinner or during a quiet moment before bed. Use these check-ins to listen actively, validate each other's feelings, and celebrate small victories, fostering an environment of trust and understanding.

- **Discussion Prompts**: Use prompts or games that encourage open-ended questions, such as "What was the best part of your day?" or "If you could travel anywhere, where would it be and why?" These prompts spark curiosity and allow family members to explore each other's dreams, perspectives, and experiences. Incorporate fun elements, like a "question jar" filled with unique prompts, to keep the activity engaging.

- **Storytelling**: Share family history, funny anecdotes, or personal experiences to build a sense of identity and connection. Storytelling not only helps children understand their roots but also instils values and life lessons. Encourage every family member to contribute their stories, creating a tradition that binds generations together and enriches family culture.

Offline Activities That Prioritise Presence

- **Game Nights**: Bring out board games, puzzles, or card games for an evening of laughter, strategy, and teamwork. Rotate who chooses the game to ensure variety and inclusivity. Incorporate themed nights, such as "retro games" or "family trivia," to keep the activity fresh and engaging. These evenings encourage healthy competition, communication, and plenty of memorable moments.

- **Learning Together**: Take a class as a family, such as cooking, dancing, or painting. Explore interests that everyone can enjoy or take turns trying activities chosen by different family members. For example, attend a pottery workshop one month and a nature photography class the next. Learning something new together not only fosters cooperation and mutual encouragement but also provides a shared sense of achievement and discovery.

- **Volunteer as a Family**: Give back to the community by participating in local events, charity drives, or environmental clean-up days. Consider adopting a long-term project, such as helping at an animal shelter or organising donations for a food bank. Volunteering cultivates a sense of purpose, empathy, and teamwork, reinforcing family values while making a positive impact on others.

Creating an Offline Routine

To make offline connections a regular part of family life, consider establishing routines that create consistency and foster meaningful interactions. Weekly tech-free nights, for example, can become a cherished tradition where family members come together to engage in board games, storytelling, or shared hobbies without the interruption of screens. Rotate activities to ensure variety and keep everyone engaged, from cooking themed dinners to organising outdoor movie nights with a projector.

Set specific times for shared activities, such as Sunday morning walks, Saturday craft sessions, or midweek family reading hours. These routines not only build stronger bonds but also create a sense of stability and anticipation within the family. Encourage everyone to actively participate in planning these activities, giving each family member a sense of ownership and excitement.

Celebrate the joy of being fully present with one another by creating rituals around these offline moments. Whether it's lighting candles during a family dinner or taking a group photo during a hike, these small touches make the time special and memorable. Reinforce the value of connection over distraction by reflecting on the experiences together and appreciating the deeper relationships that come from unplugging.

By embracing these strategies, families can create a rich, fulfilling environment where relationships thrive, traditions are built, and memories are created without the interference of screens.

Checklist *Check ✓ if you do and ✗ if you don't*

1. **Recognising Signs of Digital Overload:**

- Have I noticed changes in my child's mood, sleep patterns, or behaviour that could be linked to excessive screen time?
- Do I monitor for signs of stress, anxiety, or withdrawal related to online interactions?

2. **Promoting Healthy Screen Time:**

- Have I set appropriate screen time limits for my child's age and needs?
- Do I encourage breaks from screens, especially before bed, to protect their physical and mental health?

3. **Teaching Emotional Resilience Online:**

- Have I talked to my child about handling online negativity or comparing themselves to others on social media?
- Do I encourage them to focus on the positives of their digital experiences rather than dwelling on challenges?

4. **Balancing Online and Offline Activities:**

- Does my child have a healthy mix of digital and non-digital activities in their daily routine?
- Do I provide opportunities for them to explore offline hobbies and connect with others face-to-face?

5. **Encouraging Open Communication:**

- Have I created a safe space for my child to share their digital struggles or concerns?
- Do I regularly check in on how they feel about their online experiences?

Challenges *Check ✓ when you complete the challenges*

1. **Screen-Free Day Challenge:**

   o Designate one day each week as a "screen-free day" for the entire family.
   o Plan engaging offline activities together and reflect on how it impacts everyone's mood and interactions.

2. **Digital Mood Tracker:**

   o Work with your child to track how they feel after using different types of digital content (e.g., social media, games, educational apps).
   o Use this data to identify patterns and adjust their digital habits as needed.

3. **Mindful Media Use Exercise:**

   o Encourage your child to practise mindfulness when engaging with digital content.
   o Before they start using a device, ask: "What's my purpose for being online, and how long will I stay?"

4. **Discuss the Highlight Reel Effect:**

   o Have an open conversation about how social media often shows only the highlights of people's lives.
   o Share examples to help your child understand that comparison to these curated images can be misleading.

5. **Relaxation and Coping Techniques:**

   o Teach your child stress management techniques like deep breathing, journaling, or physical activity to balance the emotional impact of their online experiences.
   o Model these practices yourself to reinforce their importance.

Chapter 10: Building Digital Awareness and Self-Discipline

Self-discipline and digital awareness are key to managing technology responsibly in an age dominated by screens and constant connectivity. For both parents and children, cultivating these skills is essential to avoid overconsumption and ensure that technology serves as a tool for growth, learning, and connection rather than becoming a source of distraction or stress. Digital awareness empowers families to recognise how technology influences emotions, relationships, and behaviours, while self-discipline provides the framework for using it with intention and balance. This chapter provides practical strategies to establish healthy habits, foster a mindful approach to technology, and create boundaries that enable families to take control of their digital lives, ensuring technology enhances rather than detracts from their well-being.

Understanding Digital Awareness

Digital awareness involves recognising how technology impacts our emotions, behaviours, and relationships in profound and often subtle ways. Help your family identify patterns such as mindless scrolling, overreliance on notifications, or emotional reactions to online content. For example, discuss how social media "likes" or comments can influence mood and self-esteem, and how spending excessive time online might detract from other fulfilling activities.

Take the time to explain how algorithms are designed to capture attention by curating content based on past behaviour. Encourage family members to question why certain posts appear on their feed and to critically assess the intent behind advertisements or sponsored content. By fostering an understanding of these mechanisms, you empower your family to make more informed decisions about their online activities, reducing the risk of manipulation and overconsumption.

Additionally, practice self-awareness as a family by reflecting on how technology affects your overall well-being. Regularly evaluate whether digital habits align with your family's values and goals. This shared awareness fosters a culture of mindfulness, encouraging everyone to use technology in ways that enhance their lives rather than detract from meaningful connections and personal growth.

Fostering Self-Discipline

1. **Set Personal Goals**: Encourage each family member to define specific goals for their technology use, such as limiting daily screen time, avoiding devices during meals, or dedicating time to creative projects. These goals should be tailored to individual needs and regularly reviewed to ensure progress. Writing these goals down helps reinforce commitment and accountability, and creating a family "tech contract" can formalise the effort. For example, a child might commit to one hour of screen time after homework, while a parent might pledge to avoid work emails during family dinner.

2. **Create a Family Schedule**: Designate tech-free hours or activities where everyone steps away from screens. Use this time for hobbies, exercise, or meaningful conversations. Establish recurring family traditions, like Saturday morning bike rides or evening board games, to make these screen-free periods enjoyable and anticipated. Incorporate variety to ensure everyone remains engaged and invested in the activities.

3. **Practice Delayed Gratification**: Teach children the value of waiting before checking their devices. For example, encourage them to finish homework or chores before playing online games or using social media. Use small rewards, like extra story-time or a family outing, to reinforce the benefits of self-control. Explain how delaying gratification not only helps them stay focused but also cultivates resilience and patience—qualities that are valuable in every aspect of life.

By focusing on these strategies, families can foster self-discipline, creating a healthier and more balanced relationship with technology that aligns with their values and goals.

Using Technology Intentionally

- **Quality Over Quantity**: Focus on using technology for purposeful activities, such as learning new skills, creating content, or connecting with loved ones. For example, encourage children to explore educational videos, take virtual art classes, or participate in online book clubs. Set clear limits on entertainment apps and create opportunities for productive use, like researching topics of interest or developing new hobbies.

- **Mindful Consumption**: Teach children to critically evaluate online content by asking questions like, "Who created this? What is the purpose? How does it make me feel?" Help them distinguish between reliable and misleading sources by discussing the hallmarks of credible content, such as author credentials, balanced perspectives, and fact-based information. Encourage open discussions about how certain content might affect emotions or influence behaviour.

- **App Selection**: Curate apps that align with family values and promote creativity, education, or collaboration. Introduce platforms that inspire innovation, such as coding apps, language learning tools, or digital art programs. For younger children, focus on interactive apps that combine fun with skill-building. Collaborate with older children to identify and explore apps that support their interests, encouraging a proactive approach to technology use.

Establishing Digital Boundaries

- **Device-Free Zones**: Reinforce the importance of tech-free spaces in your home, such as bedrooms, dining areas, or during family outings. Create these spaces as sanctuaries for relaxation, connection, and undistracted interaction. For instance, implement a rule that family meals are tech-free, allowing everyone to focus on meaningful conversations. Add visual reminders, like signs or baskets for storing devices, to encourage adherence.

- **Screen Time Limits**: Use timers or app-based tools to manage screen usage and prevent overconsumption. Involve the whole family in setting reasonable limits based on age, needs, and activities. For example, establish a "one-hour entertainment" rule after homework or work tasks are completed. Parents can model balanced behaviour by adhering to the same limits, demonstrating the value of self-discipline.

- **Digital Detoxes**: Periodically schedule detox days where the entire family refrains from using devices, focusing instead on offline activities and relationships. Plan engaging alternatives such as outdoor picnics, board game marathons, or crafting sessions to make the detox enjoyable and anticipated. Use this time to reflect on how stepping away from screens enhances connection and well-being.

By instilling digital awareness and self-discipline, families can cultivate healthier relationships with technology and use it as a tool to enrich their lives rather than control them. This intentional approach ensures that technology supports your family's well-being and goals rather than detracting from them.

Checklist *Check ✓ if you do and ✗ if you don't*

1. **Staying Informed About Emerging Trends:**

o Do I keep up with new digital trends, apps, and platforms that my child may encounter?

o Have I educated myself about upcoming technologies like AI, virtual reality (VR), and augmented reality (AR)?

2. **Teaching Adaptability and Critical Thinking:**

o Have I discussed the importance of questioning new technologies and understanding their purpose and impact?

o Do I encourage my child to be curious and explore how technology can solve problems or foster creativity?

3. **Preparing for Ethical Technology Use:**

o Have I talked to my child about ethical issues like data privacy, digital ownership, and AI ethics?

o Do I emphasise the importance of using technology to contribute positively to society?

4. **Fostering Skills for a Digital Future:**

o Am I encouraging my child to develop skills that will be valuable in a tech-driven future, such as coding, digital design, or problem-solving?

o Do I support their participation in STEM activities or other tech-related hobbies?

5. **Balancing Optimism and Caution:**

o Have I discussed both the benefits and potential risks of future technologies with my child?

o Do I help them maintain a balanced perspective on how technology can shape their future?

Challenges *Check ✓ when you complete the challenges*

1. **Trend Exploration Activity:**
   - Spend time with your child researching one emerging technology (e.g., AI, VR, blockchain).
   - Discuss its potential uses, benefits, and challenges, and brainstorm how it might shape the future.
2. **Ethical Technology Debate:**
   - Choose a digital ethics topic (e.g., "Should AI replace human jobs?").
   - Hold a family debate to explore different perspectives and critical thinking.
3. **Future-Skills Workshop:**
   - Help your child learn a new digital skill, such as basic coding, graphic design, or robotics.
   - Use free online resources or platforms to make the experience fun and engaging.
4. **Create a "Tech Time Capsule":**
   - Work with your child to create a digital time capsule. Include screenshots, messages, or apps they use today and discuss how these might look in the future.
   - Revisit it in a few years to reflect on how technology has changed.
5. **Personal Tech Vision Exercise:**
   - Ask your child to imagine the role of technology in their life 10 years from now.
   - Encourage them to draw or write about how they see themselves using technology responsibly in the future.

What can I do to prepare my child for a future shaped by ever-changing technology? How can I teach my child to embrace technology as a tool for good while staying mindful of its challenges?

Chapter 11: Aligning Parenting Values with Technology Use

Parenting in the digital age requires aligning technology use with your family's core values, ensuring that digital habits reflect and support what matters most to your household. Technology is a pervasive force, offering both incredible opportunities and potential challenges. Without a clear strategy, it can easily conflict with the principles you aim to instil in your children. This chapter provides a comprehensive roadmap to help families define their values, create a unified approach to technology, and integrate it in ways that enhance their long-term parenting goals. By intentionally aligning digital habits with your family's core principles, you can ensure that technology serves as a tool for connection, learning, and growth rather than becoming a source of conflict or distraction.

Defining Your Family's Core Values

Begin by identifying the values that are most important to your family. These might include kindness, curiosity, responsibility, or a commitment to spending quality time together. Start by having an open discussion with all family members to explore what principles they value most. This exercise not only clarifies your shared goals but also strengthens the family's sense of unity and purpose. Reflect on how technology can either support or undermine these principles by assessing current habits and identifying areas for improvement.

For example:

- **Kindness**: Foster respectful online interactions by modelling empathy and discouraging negativity or cyberbullying. Encourage children to think before they post or comment, ensuring their actions reflect kindness and consideration.

- **Curiosity**: Use technology to inspire a love for learning by exploring educational resources, documentaries, and creative tools. For instance, engage in online courses or virtual museum tours together as a family, fostering curiosity about the world.

- **Responsibility**: Teach children to manage their screen time effectively and understand the consequences of their digital footprint. Discuss the importance of being mindful about sharing personal information online and emphasise the value of using technology responsibly to build trust and accountability.

By aligning these values with intentional technology use, families can create a digital environment that supports their principles and enhances their relationships.

Creating a Family Technology Manifesto

A family technology manifesto serves as a shared agreement outlining how your household will approach technology use. Involve all family members in creating this document to ensure it reflects everyone's needs and perspectives. By fostering collaboration, you create a sense of ownership and accountability among all family members, including children, making it more likely that the guidelines will be followed. Elements of the manifesto might include:

- **Screen Time Guidelines**: Define daily or weekly limits for different types of technology use, such as entertainment, education, and communication. Tailor these limits to fit the needs of each family member based on age, responsibilities, and other commitments. For example, younger children may have stricter limits, while teens could negotiate their own boundaries as part of a learning process.

- **Privacy and Security**: Establish rules for safeguarding personal information and maintaining online privacy. Discuss what should and shouldn't be shared online, such as addresses, school details, or private photos. Regularly review privacy settings on apps and social media platforms to ensure they align with your family's values and safety priorities.

- **Tech-Free Zones**: Specify areas or times where devices are not allowed, such as during meals, in bedrooms, or during family game nights. Enhance these tech-free zones by incorporating activities that encourage interaction, such as setting up a reading corner or a family art station.

- **Digital Etiquette and Respect**: Outline expectations for respectful and responsible online communication. This might include guidelines on how to handle disagreements online, the importance of using kind language, and the consequences of cyberbullying or inappropriate behaviour.

- **Emergency Protocols**: Include a section on what to do in case of online emergencies, such as encountering cyberbullying, phishing attempts, or inappropriate content. Ensure every family member knows who to talk to and what steps to take.

Display the manifesto prominently in your home, such as on the refrigerator or a shared bulletin board, as a reminder of your family's shared commitment to balanced and intentional technology use. Revisit and revise the manifesto regularly to adapt to new challenges or changes in technology, ensuring it remains relevant and effective in supporting your family's core values and goals.

Evaluating Your Digital Habits

Regularly assess whether your family's technology use aligns with your core values and goals. This evaluation should be an ongoing process, encouraging open dialogue and fostering mutual accountability. Use reflective questions to guide this assessment:

- **Are we spending enough time connecting face-to-face?** Evaluate whether screen use is interfering with meaningful conversations, shared activities, or quality time as a family.

- **Is technology enhancing or detracting from our goals as a family?** Consider whether digital tools are being used productively, such as for education or creative projects, versus as distractions.

- **Are we modelling the behaviours we want our children to adopt?** Reflect on your own habits, such as how often you check your phone or engage in mindful digital use, as children learn by observing their parents.

When you notice areas for improvement, involve the entire family in brainstorming solutions. Approach the discussion collaboratively to ensure buy-in from everyone. For instance:

- If screen time is cutting into outdoor play, plan regular tech-free outings like hikes, picnics, or family sports.

- If family dinners feel rushed due to device interruptions, establish a "phones-off" policy during meals and encourage everyone to share highlights from their day.

- To address overuse of social media, suggest alternative activities like starting a family project or taking up a new hobby together.

By regularly reflecting on digital habits and making adjustments as needed, your family can cultivate a healthier, more intentional relationship with technology that aligns with your shared values.

Embracing Technology with Purpose

Finally, integrate technology into your family's life in ways that amplify your values and goals. Thoughtfully incorporating digital tools can transform them into meaningful assets that enrich family life rather than detract from it. Examples include:

- **Educational Enrichment**: Explore apps and platforms that foster creativity, knowledge, and skill development. Language learning tools like Duolingo, platforms for coding such as Scratch, or apps for music composition like GarageBand can spark curiosity and encourage lifelong learning. Use these tools as opportunities for shared exploration by engaging in activities alongside your children, turning learning into a collaborative and rewarding experience.

- **Family Projects**: Collaborate on creative digital activities that bring the family together. Start a family blog to document shared experiences or milestones, create a series of home videos showcasing memorable moments, or design digital artwork together for display in your home. These projects not only develop technical and artistic skills but also strengthen familial bonds through teamwork and shared accomplishment.

- **Staying Connected**: Leverage technology to maintain and enhance relationships with extended family and friends. Regular video calls, shared photo albums, or virtual game nights can bridge physical distances and reinforce emotional connections. Encourage children to participate in these interactions, teaching them the value of maintaining meaningful relationships through digital means.

Real connections

By aligning technology use with your family's core values, you ensure that the digital world becomes a tool for growth and connection rather than a source of conflict. This intentional approach empowers your household to thrive in a connected world while staying true to what matters most. Reinforce these practices by periodically reflecting on how technology serves your family's goals, ensuring it continues to enhance your collective well-being.

Checklist *Check ✓ if you do and ✗ if you don't*

1. Defining a Digital Legacy:

o   Have I discussed with my child how their online actions and content contribute to their digital legacy?
o   Do they understand that their digital footprint reflects their values, character, and choices?

2. Teaching Long-Term Thinking:

o   Have I encouraged my child to consider how their digital activities today might impact their future (e.g., career, relationships, reputation)?
o   Do I promote a mindful approach to sharing content online, focusing on quality and intention?

3. Aligning Technology Use with Values:

o   Have I helped my child identify their core values (e.g., kindness, responsibility, creativity) and how these can guide their online behaviour?
o   Do I model value-based technology use in my own digital habits?

4. Encouraging Positive Contributions:

o   Do I inspire my child to use technology to contribute positively to their community (e.g., volunteering, sharing helpful content, supporting causes)?
o   Have I discussed how they can build connections and create opportunities through meaningful digital engagement?

5. Creating Balance:

o   Have I emphasised the importance of balancing their digital legacy with their offline achievements and relationships?
o   Do I encourage them to view their digital legacy as one part of their broader life story?

Challenges *Check ✓ when you complete the challenges*

1. **Digital Footprint Review:**

   o   Sit down with your child and review their online presence, including social media profiles, shared content, and interactions.
   o   Discuss what their current digital footprint says about them and whether it aligns with their values and goals.

2. **Legacy Vision Exercise:**

   o   Ask your child to describe how they want to be remembered online.
   o   Encourage them to create a vision statement or a set of guiding principles for their digital life.

3. **Positive Contribution Challenge:**

   o   Support your child in completing a digital project that aligns with their values (e.g., creating an educational video, supporting a charitable cause, or starting a blog about a passion).

4. **Family Digital Values Charter:**

   o   Collaborate with your child to create a family digital values charter that outlines shared goals for positive, meaningful technology use.
   o   Display the charter in a visible place as a reminder.

5. **Digital Declutter Day:**

   o   Work with your child to clean up their digital presence by deleting unnecessary or outdated content and updating privacy settings.
   o   Use this opportunity to reflect on what content best represents their values and aspirations.

Conclusion: Parenting with Purpose in the Digital Age

Parenting in the age of social media is a journey filled with unique challenges and opportunities. The digital world is ever-changing, offering tools to connect, learn, and grow, but it also presents risks that require thoughtful navigation. By understanding these challenges, modelling healthy habits, and equipping your children with the skills they need, you can guide your family toward a balanced, intentional relationship with technology.

Throughout this book, we've explored how social media influences parenting, the pressures it creates, and the tools needed to foster resilience and mindfulness in a connected world. From creating tech-free zones and setting digital boundaries to leveraging social media positively and building emotional resilience, every chapter has offered strategies to help you parent with confidence and clarity.

As you continue on this journey, remember that the ultimate goal is not perfection but progress. By aligning technology use with your family's core values and maintaining open communication, you create an environment where both children and parents can thrive. Celebrate small victories, learn from challenges, and stay flexible as you adapt to new developments in the digital landscape.

Parenting in the digital age is an opportunity to model intentionality, empathy, and purpose. By embracing these principles, you not only help your children navigate the complexities of the online world but also strengthen your family's bond in the process. Together, you can create a legacy of mindful technology use and meaningful connection that will serve your family for generations to come.

Big and Fun Tips for Parents to End on a High Note

As you close this book, here are some big and fun tips to keep in mind for navigating parenting in the digital age. Think of these as your friendly, practical reminders to carry forward:

1. Turn Off to Tune In

Set aside a "Power Down Hour" every day where the entire family puts away devices. Use this time to play, chat, or simply enjoy each other's company. Bonus points if you make it tech-free mealtime too!

2. Lead by Example

Remember, little eyes are always watching. Show your kids what balanced, mindful tech use looks like by practicing it yourself. Take breaks, stay present, and prioritise the real world.

3. Make Screen-Free Fun the Norm

Create a list of tech-free activities the whole family enjoys—like board game nights, backyard camping, or a scavenger hunt around the house. Post it on the fridge and pick one whenever the urge to scroll strikes!

4. Teach Digital Kindness

Encourage your kids to spread positivity online. Whether it's leaving a kind comment, sharing uplifting stories, or helping a friend navigate a digital issue, kindness should be their digital default.

5. Celebrate Creativity Over Consumption

Challenge your kids (and yourself!) to use tech creatively rather than passively. Create a family video project, compose music, design digital art, or start a blog. Celebrate every achievement, no matter how small.

6. Laugh Together Often

Whether it's a funny meme, a silly TikTok, or just goofing around offline, find moments to laugh together as a family. Laughter is a universal connector and a great stress reliever.

7. Stay Curious About Tech

Keep learning about the latest apps, games, and trends your kids love. Not only does it help you stay informed, but it's also a great way to connect and understand their world.

8. Remember, Progress Beats Perfection

Parenting is a marathon, not a sprint. Celebrate the wins, learn from the missteps, and know that every effort you make to parent with purpose in this digital world counts.

9. Prioritise Connection Over Perfection

It's not about perfectly managing every digital interaction—it's about fostering real, meaningful relationships. The best memories aren't measured in pixels but in laughter, love, and togetherness.

10. Make Memories, Not Metrics

Likes and followers fade, but the memories you create as a family last forever. Focus on what truly matters—shared moments of joy, discovery, and connection.

Parenting in the digital age is an adventure, and you've got this! Keep these tips handy as you navigate this journey and remember: the most valuable "shares" happen in your own home.

-END-